THE ELDERBERRY EXPERIENCE

For Your Health

STEP BY STEP GUIDE TO AN AWESOME ELDERBERRY EXPERIENCE

Why You Should Read This Book

Many people are now just discovering the benefits of elderberries. Hearing about them from friends, family, or even from health and nutrition communities, elderberries are now starting to get their time in the limelight. Far from new, however, these nutrition-packed berries have been used for centuries as a remedy and supplement.

As there are many different elderberry mixtures out there, it can be a little confusing choosing which one to try. If you are looking to add elderberries into your health routine.

This book will show you the best way to start using elderberry for its awesome benefits, both health and nutrition, there by providing you the right guardian to overcome many health and nutrition problems. Consequently improviing your overall well being...

Table of Contents

Berries are known to be some of the most nutritious things on the planet. And elderberries are one of those that you need to include in your diet. If you are wondering why, don't worry you'll know by the time you are through with this book

Elderberry is one of the most commonly used medicinal plants in the world.

If you've slogged through a cold or flu recently, you're probably familiar with elderberry. The popular virus fighter grows on a shrub (though you'll also hear it called an elderberry tree) and is a member of the Adoxaceae family. Sambucus nigra, the most typically used species, is native to Europe and North America, but it and many related species are found in temperate regions worldwide. The plant's blossoms turn to fruits called, of course, elderberries.

These edible berries are most famous for their use as an antiviral agent in medicines, and they're also used to make wine, jam, syrup, and even pie filling. The plant's flowers can be eaten or steeped as tea, and elderflower liqueur has been made for centuries.

While elderberry has prehistoric roots, its reputation as a healer may originate with the "father of medicine," Hippocrates, who called elderberry his "medicine chest" back in 400 BCE. In the Middle Ages, elderberry was called a Holy Tree, believed to have the ability to preserve health and lengthen one's life. Even greater powers have been attributed to the plant: The leaves were used to guard against witches and spirits, and people would place elderberries on windowsills to repel vampires

Traditionally, Native Americans used it to treat infections, while the ancient Egyptians used it to improve their complexions and heal burns. It's still gathered and used in folk medicine across many parts of Europe.

Today, elderberry is most often taken as a supplement to treat cold and flu symptoms

Elderberry was so named because Native American herbalists regarded it as a wise "elder" plant thanks to its ability to promote health and vitality.* Traditional Native uses include immune-boosting, wound healing, and pain-easing, as well as supporting daily regularity.* Meanwhile, in Russia and the Ukraine, it is traditional to make a tea from the tree's flowers to support respiratory health.

What Are Elderberries?

Scientifically called Sambucus berries, elderberries (also called elderflower) belong to a genus of flowering plants in the family Adoxaceae. The fruit is found in temperate to subtropical regions in the world. The elderberry tree is more widespread in the Northern Hemisphere, while in the Southern Hemisphere, it is found in parts of Australasia and South America. Several species of elderberries are cultivated not just for the fruit, but also for their ornamental leaves and flowers.

Elderberries are the fruit of the Sambucus tree. The most common type is the Sambucus nigra.

The tree has clusters of small white or cream elderflowers and bunches of small blue or black elderberries.

Native Americans and European herbalists have long used elderberries for their supposed range of health benefits. These include boosting the immune system to help the body fight off colds, flu, and other respiratory infections.

Elderberries come from a tree known as the Elder or Elderberry. It is native to North America and grows to approximately ten feet. European trees are different in that they grow taller to 25 feet. These trees have been used for several years to help with a variety of health problems. Recently, studies have proven Elderberry to be beneficial in promoting our immune system and even fighting the flu.

Sambucus nigra or Black Elderberry is the most common type of Elderberry used for medicinal purposes. Elderberry is also used for food. The flowers of the tree are used by many to make syrup, especially in Europe. This syrup is used in pancake mixes and toppings. It is also used in desserts such as pie or tarts. It is even diluted to make certain drinks.

History of Elderberries

The history of elderberries is as important to know as well.

Historically, the flowers and leaves have been used for pain relief, swelling, inflammation, to stimulate the production of urine and to induce sweating. The bark was used as a diuretic, laxative and to induce vomiting.

In folk medicine, the dried berries or juice are used to treat influenza, infections, sciatica, headaches, dental pain, heart pain and nerve pain, as well as a laxative and diuretic.

Additionally, the berries can be cooked and used to make juice, jams, chutneys, pies and elderberry wine. The flowers are often boiled with sugar to make a sweet syrup or infused into tea. They can also be eaten fresh in salads.

Historically, elderberry is known as a cure-all and has been called "the medicine chest of country people."

The Romans created hair dye from the juice. The wood of an elderberry tree is fine-grained so it polishes easily and has been used historically to make combs, toys, skewers for butchers, pegs for shoemakers and needles for weaving musical instruments.

Native Americans used the plant for healing through medicines, foods, beverages, charms, ceremonial items, inks, dyes, body paint, jewelry, hunting whistles and musical instruments.

During the 1995 Panama flu epidemic, the government employed its use to fight the flu. The berry's juice greatly reduced the time of the flu as well as the severity, thus helping end the epidemic.

There is a lot of myths surrounding the elderberry plant. In Ireland, elderberry was once considered a sacred tree. The Danish believed that the elder plant was protected by Hyldemor, the Elder Mother. It was important to ask for permission before cutting an elderberry tree or else it could bring you bad luck and misfortune. The Elder Mother was later feared as a witch with the introduction of Christianity.

Elder has both positive and negative views. The Germans and English believed that it was unlucky to bring elder wood into a house as this would bring ghosts or devils into the home. The Scotish would put elder wood above their doors and windows to protect their home from evil spirits and witches. In parts of the British Isles, they believed that bathing your eyes in the juice of the wood would allow you to see fairies.

It was believed that the cross Jesus was crucified on was made of elder wood and that the tree Judas Iscariot hung himself on was an elder. These beliefs furthered the negative view of the elderberry plant.

It is said that elder wood is best for carving steaks in vampire lore

Elderberry has a well documented history of use in folk remedies. In the Middle Ages elderberry was considered a Holy Tree, capable of restoring good health, keeping good health, and as an aid to longevity. Hippocrates referred to elderberry as "nature's medicine chest". All parts of the elderberry plant are considered a valuable healing plant in many folk and native medicine traditions (Hutchens 1991, Walker et al. 1993; Barrett et al. 1933; Clarke 1977). The flowers are used externally to aid in complexion beauty, tone and soften the skin, and lighten freckles or spots. The berry juice made into salve aids burns and scalds (Hutchens 1991). Elderberry flowers contain flavenoids and rutin, which are known to improve immune function, particularly in combination with vitamin "C." The flowers also contain tannins, which account for its traditional use to reduce bleeding, diarrhea, and congestion.

Elderberries have twice the Vitamin C of oranges and 3 times the anti-oxidants of blueberries. They are high in polyphenols and bioflavonoids. Use of the elderberry and elderflower is common and widespread in Europe. Modern science is now beginning a serious study of the plant's nutritional properties and uses.

Historical Uses

- Iroquois used a tea made from the bark of the elderberry to treat measles and headaches and used it as a strong laxative, diuretic, and a poultice for cuts.
- Cherokee used a tea made from the berries to treat boils and rheumatism and used it as a diuretic, cathartic, emetic and made a salve to treat burns.
- Leaves made into a poultice were used to stop cuts from bleeding and to treat bruises
- Bark tea was used to externally treat skin conditions such as eczema
- In Europe, extractions made from elderberry flowers and berries were used to treat colds and reduce fevers. It would also help increase bronchial secretions.
- Flowers made into a poultice have been used to ease pain and reduce inflammation
- Root was once used as an emetic and purgative, root is no longer used in modern herbal medicine
- Leaves have been used as an insect repellent and insecticide

Modern Elderberry Uses

These days, elder is most important to us because of its antibiotic compounds. We find the berry in syrups at this time of year to battle the flu. In fact, studies have found elderberry to be very effective in shortening the time of suffering and minimizing the symptoms of a bout with the flu. In lab settings we also find that elder has activity against such forgotten illnesses as mumps and measles. In fact, in the media hype over ebola, it is interesting to find that Stephen Buhner mentions in his recent book, Herbal Antibiotics, that elderberry has shown activity against this virus as well.

In modern times, elderberries played a key role in healing before the advent of antibiotics. All the parts of the plant were believed to be medicinal, including its leaves and bark, and were used in treatment for pain, as an anti-inflammatory, for toothaches, fevers, and more. The berries were also a prized food source of Native North American groups.

Nowadays, elderberry — specifically Sambucus nigra — is considered an alternative remedy for use against the common cold and flu, and it's the berries that are primarily used and given as a liquid, gummy, or capsule supplement. They're rich in flavonoids like anthocyanins, powerful plant pigments that reduce inflammation and have antiviral properties.

What Are the Potential Health Benefits of Elderberry?

There are many reported benefits of elderberries. Not only are they nutritious, but they also fight cold and flu symptoms, support heart health and fight inflammation and infections, among other benefits.

The antioxidants in elderberries contribute to most of their benefits. They boost immunity, protect the heart, and prevent cancer. The berries also improve skin and hair health. The fiber in these berries improves digestion and prevents other digestive ailments.

Boost Immunity

Several studies speak of the ability of elderberries to boost the immune system. One report published by the University of Maryland Medical Center talks about the powerful immune-boosting effects of elderberries.

The same is true with elderberry syrup as well, which increases antioxidant levels in the body and helps fight disease. The vitamins A and C in the fruit help maintain optimal health. Elderberries also offer protection against viruses that might damage cell walls.

The fruit also decreases mucus production during cold and flu, easing the symptoms. And it is one excellent remedy for the debilitating symptoms of influenza, as per a Japanese study. Elderberries boost immunity by increasing the production of inflammatory cytokines. And this way, they also help treat upper respiratory tract infections and other respiratory ailments.

Major Cold and Flu Relief

Elderberries are an excellent general immune system booster. The berries contain chemical compounds called anthocyanidins, which are known to have immunostimulant effects. Is elderberry good for a cold? Research actually shows that elderberry extract is a safe, efficient and cost-effective treatment for both cold and flu symptoms.

A 2016 study showed that elderberry supplementation can reduce the duration and symptoms of a cold in air travelers. Travelers using this herb from 10 days before travel until four to five days after arriving overseas experienced, on average, a two-day shorter duration of their colds and also a noticeable reduction in cold symptoms.

Several studies have demonstrated that elder extract is highly effective in mitigating flu-like symptoms. Specifically, the flavonoids in the elderberry extract bind to the H1N1 human influenza virus as well as the H5N1 avian influenza virus.

A 2009 study randomized patients into two groups: One group was given four doses of 175-milligram proprietary elderberry extract daily, and the other group received a placebo daily for two days. The extract-treated group showed significant improvement in most flu symptoms, while the placebo group showed no improvement or an increase in severity of symptoms. Researchers conclude that the extract is effective in controlling influenza symptoms.

Another study published in the Journal of International Medical Research showed that when the extract is used within the first 48 hours of the onset of flu symptoms, it shortens the duration of flu symptoms by an average of four days.

Black elderberry extracts and flower infusions have been shown to reduce the severity and length of influenza.

Commercial preparations of elderberry for the treatment of colds come in various forms, including liquids, capsules, lozenges and gummies.

One study of 60 people with influenza found that those who took 15 ml of elderberry syrup four times per dayshowed symptom improvement in two to four days, while the control group took seven to eight days to improve.

Another study of 64 people found that taking 175-mg elderberry extract lozenges for two days resulted in significant improvement in flu symptoms, including fever, headache, muscle aches and nasal congestion, after just 24 hours.

Furthermore, a study of 312 air travelers taking capsules containing 300 mg of elderberry extract three times per day found that those who got sick experienced a shorter duration of illness and less severe symptoms.

During flu season you know you need to wash your hands constantly, but you may also try elderberry.

Improve Digestive Health

Though research is limited here, elderberries, like most fruits, are good sources of fiber and can enhance digestion. The fiber in the fruit can also treat other digestive issues like constipation, stomach upset, gas, and bloating.

Can Help Prevent Cancer

Scientists from numerous parts of the world had used elderberries in cancer treatment, with much success. This can be attributed to the quercetin in elderberries – whose therapeutic effects can stimulate the immune system and aid the treatment.

Other studies show that elderberries can also treat prostate cancer. The berries are known to inhibit a biochemical process called hedgehog signaling, which has been linked to cancer.

Eldible berry extracts like elderberry extract are rich in anthocyanins and have been shown to have a broad spectrum of therapeutic, pharmacologic and anti-carcinogenic properties. Laboratory studies specifically indicate that the elderberry has some chemopreventive properties. A chemopreventive inhibits, delays or reverses cancer formation.

One study published in the Journal of Medicinal Food compared the anticancer properties of European and American elderberry fruits. European elderberry (Sambucus nigra) is known for its medicinal use and contains anthocyanins, flavonoids and other polyphenolics, which all contribute to the high-antioxidant capacity of its berries. American elderberry (Sambucuscanadensis) has not been grown or promoted as a medicinal plant like its European relative.

This study took extracts of both berries and tested them to access anticancer potential. Both extracts demonstrated significant chemopreventive potential. Additionally, the American elder extract showed inhibition of ornithine decarboxylase, which is an enzyme marker related to the promotion stage of cancer formation. These findings indicate the potential as a natural cancer treatment option.

Enhance Heart Health

Given that they are rich in potassium (and also they have a great potassium to sodium ratio), elderberries can help regulate blood pressure. They ensure the blood vessels relax. Also, a high potassium diet is known to reduce the strain on the heart. Studies have shown that individuals taking a high amount of potassium (and by this, we don't mean excess) had a 49 percent less risk of death by ischemic heart disease.

Some sources also say that elderberries can help regulate cholesterol levels and even boost circulation (and this offers good exercise to the heart and keeps it in shape).

Elderberries also contain beneficial compounds called anthocyanins, which protect the inner layer of the blood vessels from oxidative stress. This protects the cells from inflammatory stressors, ultimately improving circulation and cutting the risk of heart disease.

Although the studies in this field have found mixed results, there is research suggesting that elderberry extract may improve cardiovascular health. When mice with high cholesterol and HDL cholesterol dysfunction were given anthocyanin-rich black elderberry extract, they had a reduction in hepatic cholesterol levels with improvement in HDL function. This may be due to the presence of anthocyanins, which are polyphenols found in elderberry that have demonstrated antioxidant and anti-inflammatory activities.

And another study found that elderberry extract may have beneficial effects on high blood pressure. When polyphenols extracted from the elderberry plant were given to rats with hypertension, in combination with renin inhibitors, they reduced arterial pressure. Researchers suggest that using polyphenols, like those found in elderberry, to lower blood pressure may also help to reduce the side effects of antihypertensive agents and improve patient quality of life.

Elderberry may have positive effects on some markers of heart and blood vessel health.

Studies have shown elderberry juice may reduce the level of fat in the blood and decrease cholesterol. In addition, a diet high in flavonoids like anthocyanins has been found to reduce the risk of heart disease.

However, another study in mice with high cholesterol found that a diet including black elderberry reduced the amount of cholesterol in the liver and aorta but not the blood

Further studies found that rats fed with foods containing polyphenols extracted from elderberry had reductions in blood pressure and were less susceptible to organ damage caused by high blood pressure

Furthermore, elderberries may reduce levels of uric acid in the blood. Elevated uric acid is linked to increased blood pressure and negative effects on heart health .

What's more, elderberry can increase insulin secretion and improve blood sugar levels. Given that type 2 diabetes is a major risk factor for heart and vascular disease, blood sugar control is important in preventing these conditions.

A study found that elderberry flowers inhibit the enzyme α-glucosidase, which may help lower blood sugar levels. Also, research on diabetic rats given elderberry showed improved blood sugar control.

Despite these promising results, a direct reduction in heart attacks or other symptoms of heart disease has not yet been demonstrated, and further studies in humans are needed.

Can Help Treat Diabetes

Reports shows that elderberries can help lower blood sugar levels, aiding diabetes treatment. However, studies are limited in this regard, and I'll advise you to talk to your doctor first.

Both the elder flower and the berry have traditionally been used to treat diabetes. Research has confirmed that extracts of elderflower stimulate glucose metabolism and the secretion of insulin, lowering blood sugar levels.

Research evaluated black elderberry's insulin-like and insulin-releasing actions in vitro. The study found that an aqueous extract of elder significantly increased glucose transport, glucose oxidation and glycogenesis without any added insulin. What is glycogenesis, and why is it important? Glycogenesis is the process by which excess sugar is cleared out of the bloodstream and into your muscles and liver, which helps maintain normal blood sugar.

And a 2017 animal study published in the International Journal of Molecular Sciences suggests that elderberries can serve as a potential source of bioactive compounds for formulations that are used for the management of diabetes. Researchers found that both lipophilic and polar extracts of elderberry lowered insulin resistance in wistar rats with type 2 diabetes

Strengthen Bones

The calcium, iron, and potassium in the berries are known to strengthen bones and increase bone mineral density, cutting the risk of osteoporosis as a result.

Additionally, the anthocyanins in the berries might prevent bone loss in certain cases. As of now, we need more clarity on this. But do consult your doctor.

Can Aid Weight Loss

Just like most fruits, elderberries are rich in fiber. And fiber, as we know, improves satiety and can aid weight loss. This has been proven by a German study as well – where participants taking elderberry juice enriched with elderberry flower and the extracts saw a significant improvement in weight regulation.

Improve Skin And Hair Health

Infused with innate anti-aging and free radical fighting properties, elderberries keep your skin radiant for longer periods. Furthermore, they also act as a natural detoxifying agent and help prevent distressing skin conditions like breakouts, boils, and scars.

The anthocyanins in elderberries (the compounds that give them their characteristic red color) were found to give a natural boost to your skin's health. This compound also protects against skin damage. In fact, distilled elderberry flower water is known to restore skin health and lighten the freckles. Applying the fruit extract can also reduce inflammation and bruising. The extract can help treat herpes as well. The antioxidants in the berry can fight the herpes virus and give relief.

The berries work great for your hair as well. You can take some elderflower oil (you should be getting it in the market) and mix it with some of your other favorite oils. Apply on the problem areas of your scalp. The serum can treat split ends, problematic hairlines, and might even encourage hair growth.

Elderberry has made its way into cosmetic products, and for good reason. Its bioflavonoids and antioxidants, along with its high vitamin A content, make it awesome for skin health. Researchers suspect that a compound found in the elderberry could give a natural boost to skin.

A compound found in elderberry, called anthocyanin, has proven to have anti-inflammatory and antioxidant properties. Researchers found that this compound may improve the skin's structure and condition.

Can Boost Vision Health

Being rich in vitamins A and B6, elderberries can help prevent serious vision ailments like glaucoma and macular degeneration. The antioxidant activity of elderberries also helps ensure vision health in the long run.

Help Treat Urinary Tract Infections

Though there is very limited research on this, certain sources note that infusions of elderberry juice can help reduce inflammation in the urinary tract and treat urinary tract infections.

Fight Inflammation

Numerous studies talk about the anti-inflammatory properties of elderberries. In fact, the berries have even been used to treat eye inflammation.

Another study states how anthocyanins in elderberries can help fight inflammation . They achieve this by fighting oxidative stress.

Sinus Infection Aid

With elderberry's anti-inflammatory and antioxidant properties, it makes sense that it can help sinus issues. A sinus infection is a condition in which the cavities around the nasal passages become inflamed, and this antiviral herb has promise as a sinus infection natural remedy.

A study conducted by the Institute of Complementary Medicine's Department of Internal Medicine at the University Hospital in Zurich, Switzerland examined the use of a proprietary product, Sinupret, which contains elderberry flowers. The researchers used Sinupret to treat bacterial sinusitis along with an antibiotic (doxycycline or vibramycin) and a decongestant. People who took the combination did better compared to those who did not take Sinupret at all.

Improve Brain Health

One study talks about how the anthocyanins in berries (including elderberries) can help treat cognitive impairment and the resultant conditions like Alzheimer's.

Elderberries are also replete with quercetin, which is an important flavonoid critical for brain health. Quercetin reduces the harmful inflammation at a cellular level. It also activates the mitochondria in your cells – which are powerhouses that boost cell health.

That's with the benefits. But there are other ways you can use elderberries.

Ease Allergies

The flowers of the elder plant are known to be an effective herbal allergy remedy. Since allergies involve an overreaction of the immune system as well as inflammation, elderberry's ability to improve the immune system and calm inflammation can help provide allergy relief.

Some herbalists put black elder flower on the list of most effective herbs used for treating hay fever-like symptoms. It can be used for allergies on its own or in combination with other herbs. Elderflower is also said to act as a detoxification aid by enhancing liver function.

Top Elderberry Types to Grow in Your Backyard

You can certainly propagate existing plants – especially if you are fortunate to have them growing wild in your region. But many gardeners choose to buy proven varieties from nurseries and garden centers.

I am identifying few of the favorite cultivars of elderberry

BLACK LACE ELDERBERRY

This unique version of the common Sambucus plant has dark leaves that appear lacey throughout the growing season. When the flowers come on, you'll be delighted to find that they are pink!

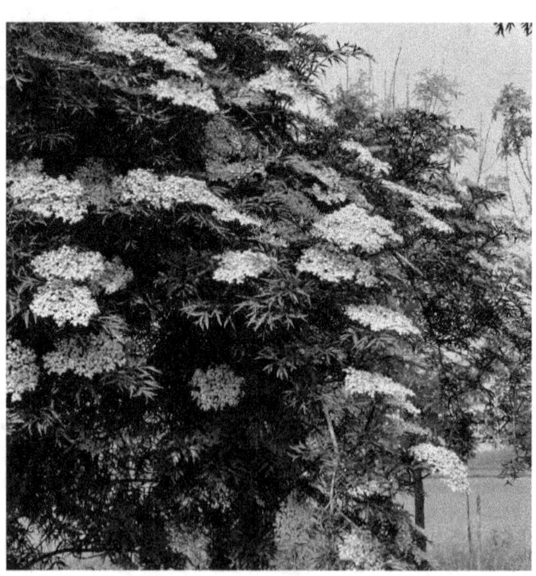

This plant also produces the same versatile berry as other more common varietals.

Many gardeners find that the plant's need for moisture makes it a perfect rain garden addition.

Black Lace works in almost any soil except extremely dry ones. It love wet soils and is great in a rain garden setting. It only reaches to 8' high so it can fit into any garden, but you can prune it to any height you like. It makes a great hedge or foundation plant. Try it as a specimen plant or small tree

The Black Lace variety thrives in US Hardiness Zones 4-7

ADAMS ELDERBERRY

This native cultivar of Sambucus canadensis goes by the common name "Adams." It is one of the most common elderberries grown in North America and is similar to those found growing wild.

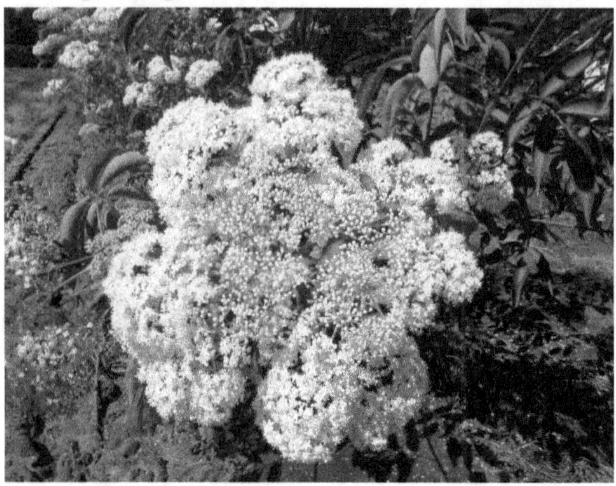

The signature white flowers, and large clusters of dark purple fruits, make it easily identifiable as a beautiful yard accent.

At full height, this beautiful bush can reach between 6 and 10 feet tall. It will thrive in USDA Hardiness Zones 3-9.

BLUE ELDERBERRY

This plant is native to the western United States, Mexico, and the West Coast

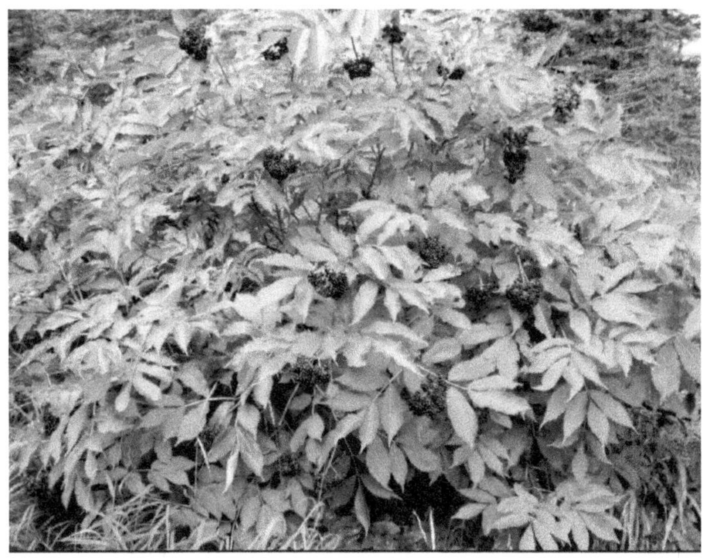

With large, powdery-blue berries, it can sometimes be confused for a form of blueberry. The fruits on this stunning bush are known for having a rich flavor.

This blue variety differs from others in that it grows best from seed. It thrives in warmer regions, and therefore is best suited for growing zones 3 through 10

LEMON LACE ELDERBERRY

Also known as Lemony Lace, this is a very hardy and showy plant that has feathery, light-colored leaves. S. racemose produces red fruits in the fall, after the white flower bunches have died away.

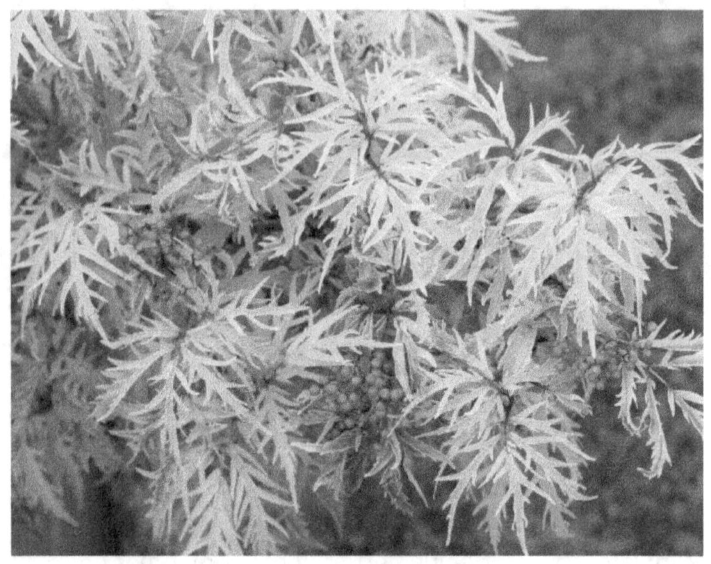

Amazingly deer-, cold-, and wind-resistant, it does well in full sun and is a prized plant in the northern United States. It's versatile enough, however, to thrive in partial shade in southern states as well.

Plant in zones 3-7 and enjoy this adaptable plant with its uniquely beautiful chartreuse color. Please note that some experts cautions against eating S. racemose cultivars, i.e. those with red berries.

YORK ELDERBERRY

Another old-style elderberry, this one is reported to have the largest berries and the highest fruit yield

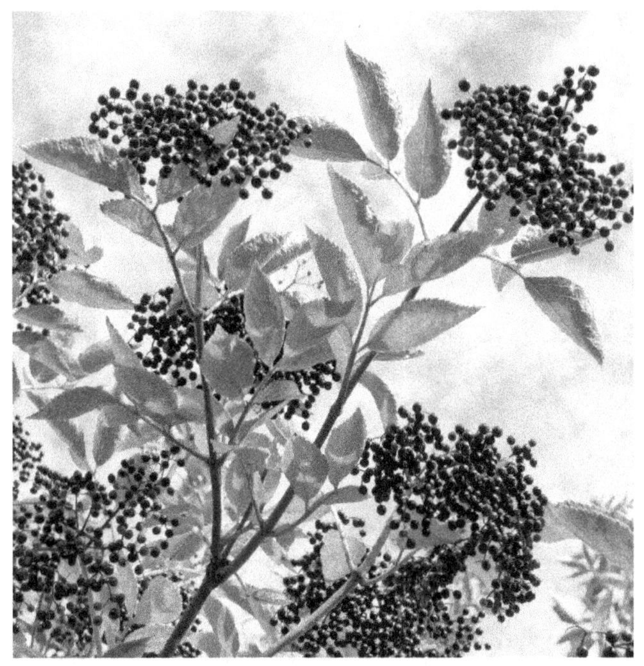

This resilient breed is also cold tolerant, making it a perfect choice for zones 3-9. Many growers use it as a natural fencing solution, since bushes can grow up to 12 feet tall.

Fall brings about a beautiful color change in this plant. Foliage becomes bright red before dropping off for the winter

EUROPEAN RED ELDERBERRY

This imported beauty has amazing cherry-red fruits in the fall, and light green, feathery foliage makes it a beautiful yard accent.

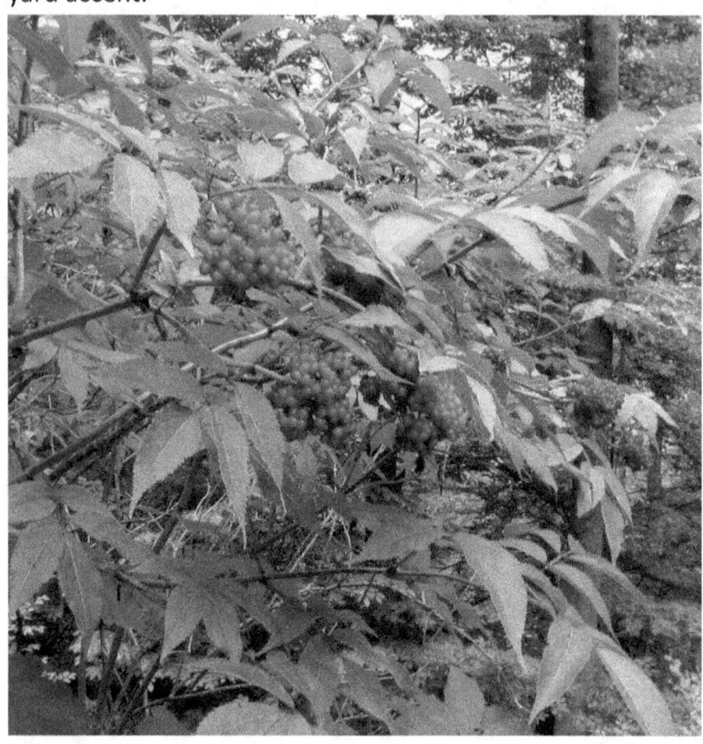

Owners of the plant are usually stunned by how attracted birds and pollinators are to the large, showy flowers. Butterflies are almost always nearby!

Propagate in the spring for a full-grown, eye-catching bush within two to three years. It has the potential to reach up to 20 feet tall in growing zones 3-8. Please note that some experts caution against eating varieties with red berries, and many favor black varieties since red ones tend to be pungent and bitter, with many seeds.

BLACK BEAUTY ELDERBERRY

A new import from Europe, this variety has very dark leaves, pinkish blooms, and a unique lemon scent.

It is best suited for US growing zones 4-7 and prefers moist or even wet growing conditions.

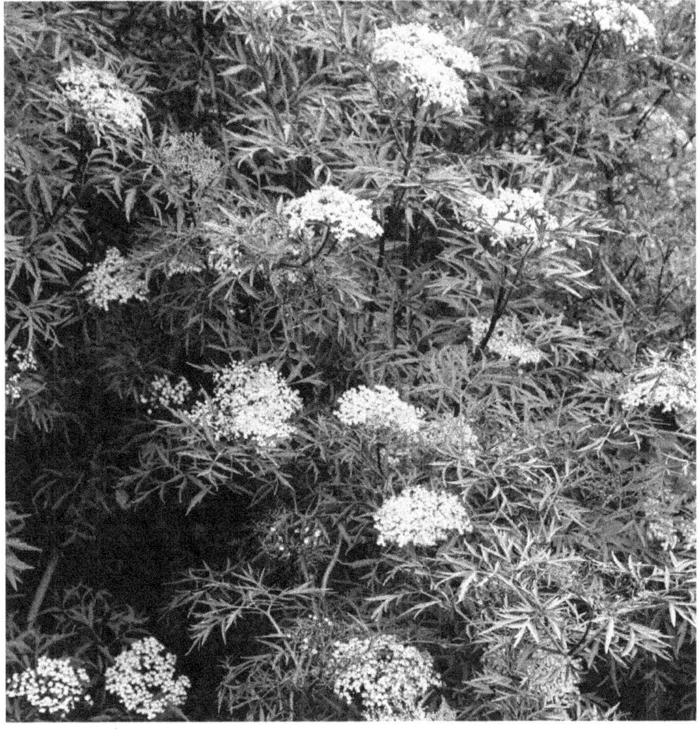

A smaller elderberry breed, this plant will grow to no more than 6 feet at maturity, but responds well to pruning.

Like other elderberries, it produces luscious fruits that have become popular for making delicious wines. Buy two to ensure proper cross-pollination.

Care and Planting of Elderberries for Every Garden

If you have room for only one edible plant, consider the elderberry. This arching eight-foot tall shrub is easy to grow, anchors the mixed border with its bold compound foliage and flowers, and of course, provides glorious clusters of shiny, dark purple berries.

Elderberries come in a variety of cultivars and species. The American species is Sambucus canadensis. Look for this species if you want to harvest as many berries as possible. 'Nova' and 'York' are the two cultivars that set the biggest crops. Although these varieties are self-fruitful, you'll get a bigger crop with two plants because they cross-pollinate one another for larger yields. Elder flowers are used for fritters, they're great for bouquets, and the berries make the most intensely colored claret wine you'll ever see. You can eat the berries off the shrub, but they're better in jams, syrups and pies. Throw some berries into a peach pie for a special summertime treat.

The European species is Sambucus nigra. This species is parent to some spectacular new hybrids, including the 2006 introduction 'Black Lace.' The purple-black foliage is deeply imbricated and looks like a cutleaf Japanese maple. The massive pink flower heads that appear in late Spring confound the most expert gardeners. Like the American varieties, 'Black Lace' is self-fertile, but benefits from the presence of another variety nearby for cross-pollination. Another purple-leafed European cultivar is 'Black Beauty.'

This plant is similar to 'Black Lace' in coloration, but the leaves are oval. The showy drooping berry clusters on both varieties must be cooked before eating. They're great for jams and syrups. A S. nigra cultivar called 'Pulverulenta' has pale green leaves mottled with creamy white. It's a beautiful shrub for a woodland garden. The flowers are typical white elder cymes that are perfectly showcased by the marbled foliage. You'll get enough berries to satisfy birds, but not enough for jam or pie making. Try growing the beautiful green-white Clematis florida alba semi-plena into the branches of this variegated shrub for an extra visual kick.

Another species in the elderberry family is Sambucus racemosa. Native to the northern latitudes of North America, Europe and Asia, this elderberry bears red berries that are best left to the birds.

If you want to attract wildlife, elderberries are a great choice. Butterflies are frequent visitors to elder flowers, and elderberries are a favorite with many birds. Woodpeckers, bluebirds, cedar waxwings, orioles and grosbeaks will choose elderberries over anything else in your garden.

Elderberries have no diseases to speak of, they're very adaptable to a variety of soil conditions, moisture levels and sunlight, and deer tend to leave them alone. They grow well in Zones 4-9. You can prune them back every year after fruiting to keep them in check. And don't forget to bring in branches of flowers and berries for striking bouquets.

Step by step guide to planting

If you want to grow this plant in your garden, you need to know that caring for it in the first years of its life is a little more specific - it prefers moist soil and you don't have to expect fruits until its second year. Better plant two or more shrubs near each other to make the cross-pollination easier

Step 1: Find Your Elderberry Bush

If you know of a friend or neighbor that has one, ask them if you can get a clipping. If not, chances are good that if you ask around someone will know where to get one. You might post on Facebook to see if anyone in your extended community has a bush they'd be willing to let you take a clipping from.

If you have difficulty finding elderberry bushes in your area, you can order from a Farm. You can order for three different types of elderberry cuttings to maximize fruitfulness. "Cross pollination is not required to produce fruit, but flowers that are cross-pollinated will produce larger fruit—it is beneficial to have two cultivars of elderberry in close proximity." In other words, if you plant two different varieties within 60 feet of each other you increase the fruitfulness of both.

When I first started looking for elderberries in the wild, I was terrified I'd confuse it with Pokeberry or Water Hemlock, which are poisonous. Fortunately, if you know what to check for they are VERY easy to tell apart.

Identifying elderberries from water hemlock:

The most common confused questions I hear on identification are about elderberries and the water hemlock. the two species don't look alike at all. Generally said elderberry fruit is edible, the entire water hemlock is deadly. Indeed, many call water hemlock the most deadly plant in North America. Learning to identify the two is very important.

The Elderberry, Sambucus canadensis, is a shrub with bark, to ten feet or more. Woody. Its blossom is a dense flattop. It produces, locally, black berries about BB size. It has opposite compound leaves, feathery. Most of the veins on the leaf either fade after leaving the midrib or terminate at the tip of the teeth, not in the notches. If you have a #10 magnifying glass you can see tiny veins terminating at the tips of the teeth. Occasionally an elderberry vein will terminate at a notch, but it is uncommon

The Water Hemlock is herbaceous, two to seven feet. It has a green main stem with purple splotches, or is entirely dusky purple particularly when young. The sectioned, hollow stem has vertical grooves on the outside. It produces a fire cracker-like explosion white blossom that made up of many smaller umbrella-like blossoms. Those produce seeds, not fruit. It has alternating, compound leaves, coarse, toothy. On individual leaves most, not all, but most of the veins clearly terminate between the teeth, in the notches.

Let's also talk about habitat. Both elderberries and water hemlock are associated with water. But there are some differences: Elderberries can tolerate more dry areas and Water Hemlock can grow in water. If you are in a dry area that is dry most of the time and you think you have one or the other it will probably be an elderberry. If you have damp ground it can be either. If it is standing water most of the time it will probably be water hemlock. Season also counts. Elderberries are year round locally. Water Hemlock can die back in the winter.

Elderberries are shrubs. They are woody. They have bark. The bark is green and smooth when very young with occasional white dots that are actually lenticels, which is one way the plant exchanges gasses. With time and height the elderberry develops a familiar looking bark, smooth and brown. Now the lenticels are corky lumps. On much older plants the bark will become vertically furrowed. The inner core of the trunk and branches — the pith — is soft and can be easily reamed out. Not a long-lived plant, just a few years, it can grow to about four inches through. When it dies and dries it leaves a vertical standing small dead tree. The dead wood breaks easily and burns well.

The Water Hemlock is herbaceous, read not woody. It does not have bark. It has nodes, which are swellings where leaves attach or used to attach. The main stem has vertical groves in it and is hollow. It is often streaked with purple, or is splotched with purple. It is usually at least purple at the nodes and sometimes young plants can be entirely dusky purple. Ocassionally the entire older plant will be purple. A stem that is an inch through would be a large water hemlock. The plant is hairless. When crushed it can have a pleasant liquorish or anise scent, or it can also smell like mouse urine. Remember it is deadly and can kill in virtually minutes. The toxicity decreases vertically with the roots the most toxic and the seeds the least. Taste is not a warning sign in that those who have eaten the roots raw or cooked said they were flavorful and very enjoyable. Depending upon the size of the individual, the amount consumed and which parts consumed death will occur in 15 minutes to a little over two hours. This is not the hemlock given to Socrates which was a gentle species. This species produces severe pain and convulsions, torturing its victim horribly until death.

The leaves of both species are different, not only from a distance but close up as well. The veins of the elderberry leaf either fade as they reach the edge of the leaf or terminate at the tip of the teeth. You may need a small magnifying class to see that. The veins are most prominent as they leave the light-colored midrib. Also note that the teeth are quite small, like the edge of a small serrated steak knife

The veins of the water hemlock are quite different. The veins of the water hemlock clearly terminate BETWEEN the larger teeth of the leaf. See arrows to right. There is no ambiguity. The veins end between the teeth. Even when a vein splits the split ends go to the notches, not to the tips of the leaf. There may be an occasional exception but the trend of the majority is very clear. You will note that while each species' leaf has an acute tip (pointed) the elderberry leaf is round near the tip whereas the water hemlock leaf is not.

The elderberry is not without its dangers as well. The wood is toxic and has poisoned folks who have made whistles out of the green wood. Unripe elderberry fruit is toxic and the ripe fruit bothers some people. The ripe fruit is better used dried, cooked or made into wine or jelly than consumed raw

Once you've identified your elderberry bush, you can cross-check it by cutting it down the center. Elderberry has a hard, woody stem with a soft center describes as "like styrofoam."

Step 2: Gather Your Elderberry Cuttings

While the bush is dormant, usually January through March, use pruning shears to cut a 8-9 inch section of elderberry cane. (That's the hard, woody stem I mentioned earlier.) You want the cut to be slanted to improve the canes ability to draw up moisture.

it's best to "focus on stems that are very green in spring, those that are sturdy but thinner than the older canes at the center of the clump . . . Choose ones that are about as big around as your little finger and located on the edges of the thicket."

Step 3: Encourage Root Growth

And by encourage, I don't mean grab your pom poms and cheer. (Though you can totally do that if you want to.)

There are two main ways to help your trimmings establish roots.

WATER METHOD

Place your trimmings (cut side down) in a mason jar and add water until they are halfway submerged. Place the jar in a sunny area for 6-8 weeks, changing the water often.

Spritz with water occasionally – elderberry bushes love a humid environment. Roots grown in water are more fragile than ones grown in soil, so wait until they look sturdy before transferring. When they're ready and there is not risk of freezing temperatures, plant the elderberry bush into quality soil – the kind that you'd use in a vegetable garden – with good drainage.

SOIL METHOD

Place your trimmings (cut side down) in a mason jar and add water until they are halfway submerged. Allow them to soak for 12-24 hours and then transfer them to pots filled with good, organic soil. (Again, the kind you would use in a vegetable garden.) Keep the pots moist so that the cuttings don't dry out. They need a humid environment to encourage growth, so either:

Place them in a greenhouse

Place a plastic bag over the top to trap moisture and create a greenhouse-like effect, then set the pot in a sunny area.

The trimmings will send out leaves and then grow roots – it can take six to twelve weeks to see significant root growth according to Rodger. Once it reaches the 6-8 week mark, gently tug on the cutting to assess root development. Once they're well established and there is not risk of freezing temperatures, plant the elderberry cane (roots intact) into the soil.

Step 4: Planting Your Elderberry Bush

"Transplant the elderberry cutting into the landscape in the spring following rooting. Pick a spot that gets full sun or part shade, with humus rich soil and good drainage. Dig a planting hole and place the new elderberry shrub into the soil with the base of the stem level with the soil line."

Elderberry bushes can grow to be 6-8 feet wide, so space your bushes out by 6-10 feet

Step 5: Make Elderflower Lemonade!

Seriously, this is a step. During your elderberry bushes' first season you want to pinch off the flowers so that the elderberry can devote it's energy to developing a strong root system. Use them to make syrup, tea or lemonade.

Next season you'll be harvesting elderberries! What's growing in your garden this year?

After you have done your elderberry planting, you should cultivate once in a while very carefully. You do not want to disturb the roots. Use mulch where necessary to prevent weed growth, and pluck those weeds that manage to sneak through. When growing elderberries, remember that the bushes require about 25 mm of water a week. Therefore, if summertime comes and you find that you are running into periods of no rain, be sure to water them often. The first two years after planting elderberry bushes, you should let them grow wildly. Do not prune and do not bother picking the berries. After that, you can prune the elderberry bushes in the early spring by cutting them back and removing all the dead areas. This way, the bushes will grow and produce a lot of berries for you. Right around mid-August and mid-September, there is a five to 15-day ripening period. Be sure to pick them before the birds do, and enjoy.

Harvesting and Preparing the Fruits

If you ask me, the most labor-intensive part of owning an elderberry is harvesting the fruit. Removing the berries from the plant is easy. Everything after that, however, takes some skill.

You'll want to harvest when the berries are as dark purple, or even as black, as you can imagine they will get. They should be very soft and juicy.

If they appear shriveled, like a raisin, you've waited too long.

Picking them before the birds do is tough. If you have a good number of berries in clusters that are close to being ready, you may go ahead and get all of them.

It's impossible to pick individual berries, so you must eyeball the group and go for a good percentage of ripe ones when making your decision. Again, if almost all are ripe, the birds will probably get to them by the next day.

Using a good pair of pruning shears, cut the entire cluster just under the base of where the fruits begin. I put them into a 5-gallon plastic bucket from the hardware store and take all of them home at once.

PREPARING THE FRUITS

Whether you plan on canning for jelly and jam, making a pie, or concocting a tincture to fight colds and flu, this process is necessary for any use of the fruits.

If bugs are crawling all over your fruits, you can allow the clusters to soak in water for a few hours and then use right away. Or, you can wait a day and do this easy freezing method:

1. Rinse the clusters of berries and lay flat on a towel to drain.

2. Place each cluster on a parchment-lined cookie sheet. Place the entire sheet into the freezer for at least 24 hours.

3. Once the fruits are frozen, remove them and place into a plastic gallon storage bag.

4. Hit the bag gently against a counter until you hear all of the little frozen fruits rattling around in the bag.

Separate the stems, which should be mostly in one piece, from the fruits. Voila!

If you don't like the idea of freezing, lack storage space, or want to use the fruits right away, you can use a fork to remove the fruits from the stems.

Starting at the thickest part of the berry bunch, scrape along each stem, pulling the berries with it as you go.

Note that you'll also gather quite a bit of stemmy material with this method. Be sure to follow it up with a triple rinse in a fine mesh strainer afterwards.

How to Dry and Store

Elder has a long history of being used in a variety of home-made recipes, medicines and cosmetics, with the Elderberries making excellent wine. They can also be used in pies, cakes and jams, along with cold and flu remedies. So how can you make the most of this free bounty?

If making Elderberry wine, fresh Elderberries are really the only way to go. You will want to use them as soon as possible, storing in a cool, dark place until use. If you are planning on using them for pies and other tasty delights, or even for general storage for later use, you will want to dry the berries. Regardless of how you intend to use them, it is worth remembering that you need to remove all stalks before use, otherwise they can taint the finished product with a bitter taste.

When collecting the Elderberries you will want to cut them at the main stalk, rather than trying to tear or pinch it. As with Elderflowers, it is best to pick the berries when they are dry, so avoid picking after rain or first thing in the morning when covered in dew. Remember to only take what you will use, taking too much and throwing them away is just sacrilege.

Elderberries can be dried a couple of ways - with time and patience or quickly in the oven.

The time and patience way includes hanging them by the stalks to air dry for a period of ten days. Make sure you cover with a paper bag, with air holes pierced in it - this will catch any that may fall during the drying process. You can hold the bag in place with an elastic band.

A much quicker way to dry Elderberries is to remove all the stalks and spread them on trays for cooking in a warm oven. You will need to preheat the oven to 50oC (or less) and leave them in there for 7-14 minutes. Be careful not to overcook them - you want them to resemble raisins. You then need to remove them from the oven and leave until completely cold.

How to Use Elderberry

Elderberry can be purchased in many forms at your local farm or health store or online.

Ways to Consume Elderberry

- Tea

- Wine

- Juice

- Jelly and jams

- Syrup

- Ointments

- Astringent

- Infusions

- Sprays

- Lozenges

- Pills

- Liquid

- Powder

- Capsules

When it comes to colds, flu and upper respiratory issues, elderberry syrup is very popular. There are high-quality brands readily available for purchase, or you can try making your own.

Elderberry tea is another great option. You can either buy teabags or you can purchase dried berries or flowers and make a tea by combining 1 tablespoon of berries or flowers with 8 ounces of water.

Not a fan of hot teas? Then you can try elderberry juice, which is sweet, tart and refreshing. Just watch out that you don't purchase one that has too much added sugar.

Health Risks and Side Effects

What are the side effects and health risks of elderberry?

While elderberry has many promising potential benefits, there are also some dangers associated with its consumption.

The bark, unripe berries and seeds contain small amounts substances known as lectins, which can cause stomach problems if too much is eaten.

In addition, the elderberry plant contains substances called cyanogenic glycosides, which can release cyanide in some circumstances. This is a toxin also found in apricot seeds and almonds.

There are 3 mg of cyanide per 100 grams of fresh berries and 3–17 mg per 100 grams of fresh leaves. This is just 3% of the estimated fatal dose for a 130-pound (60-kg) person.

However, commercial preparations and cooked berries do not contain cyanide, so there are no reports of fatalities from eating these. Symptoms of eating uncooked berries, leaves, bark or roots of the elderberry include nausea, vomiting and diarrhea.

There is one report of eight people falling ill after drinking the juice from freshly picked berries, including the leaves and branches, from the S. mexicana elder variety. They experienced nausea, vomiting, weakness, dizziness, numbness and stupor.

Luckily, toxic substances found in the berries can be safely removed by cooking. However, the branches, bark or leaves should not be used in cooking or juicing.

If you are collecting the flowers or berries yourself, ensure that you have correctly identified the plant as American or European elderberry, as other types of elderberry may be more toxic. Also, be sure to remove any bark or leaves before use.

If you were to come across an elderberry plant, you'd be best served by cooking the berries. The bark, leaves, seeds, and unripe fruit may cause cyanide poisoning when ingested. Side effects of uncooked berries include nausea or vomiting. Luckily, cooking does eliminate their toxicity. But watch the amount: When cooked berries "are consumed in amounts usually found in foods," they're likely safe, but don't go overboard. Finally, it's only the blue and purple berries that are edible. The red berries that dot other elderberry plant species are toxic. Don't eat them.

If you're being treated for certain medical conditions you may need to stay away from elderberries. Always talk to your doctor first, especially if you're on any prescription medication, such as blood pressure medications (elderberries may lower blood pressure, compounding the effect of the drug), on chemotherapy (they may increase the risk of side effects), or if you have been diagnosed with diabetes (they may alter insulin secretion). These are just a few of the conditions that elderberry may interact with, so it's critical that your doctor knows everything you're taking, including natural supplements.

If you're pregnant, you may consider turning to elderberry rather than conventional medications, but it's not known yet if it's safe. When researchers reviewed the literature on elderberry, they found that there weren't enough clinical trials on the safety of elderberry in pregnancy. And while some trials have shown that elderberry is effective against the flu, that data is culled from a small number of people, and more research is needed. As it stands, researchers say, doctors should not tell their pregnant patients to take elderberry for upper respiratory infections

Elderberry Recipes

Elder Flower Fritters

Elder flower fritters are truly a gift from the heavens. Gather some of the clusters of the elderberry flowers.

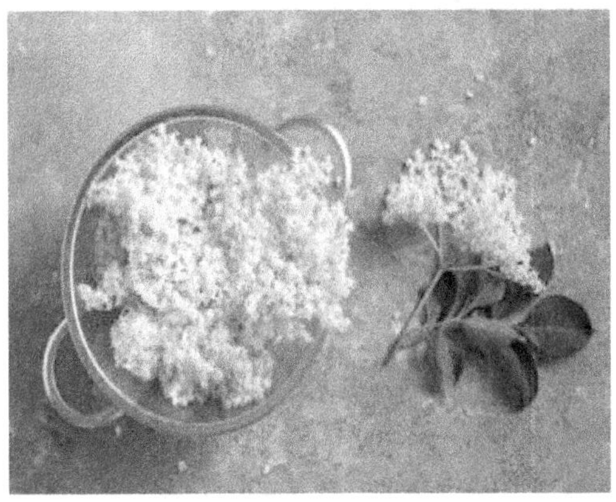

Snip off the greenish branches connected to the flowers but keep them in a bunch ready for making fritters.

Ingredients:

- 2 cups flour

- 1 tablespoon baking powder

- 1 teaspoon salt

- 2 eggs

- 1 teaspoon vanilla

- 2/3 cup milk

• Several bunches of creamy white elder flowers

Directions:

Mix all batter ingredients together except the elder flowers until you've got a smooth and even batter. Dip flowers in batter and lightly fry in a skillet until golden brown. You could also try sprinkling the elder flowers directly into the batter for a lacy treat. I've cooked them both ways and they are both equally satisfying. Enjoy with elderberry syrup

Basic Elderberry Syrup

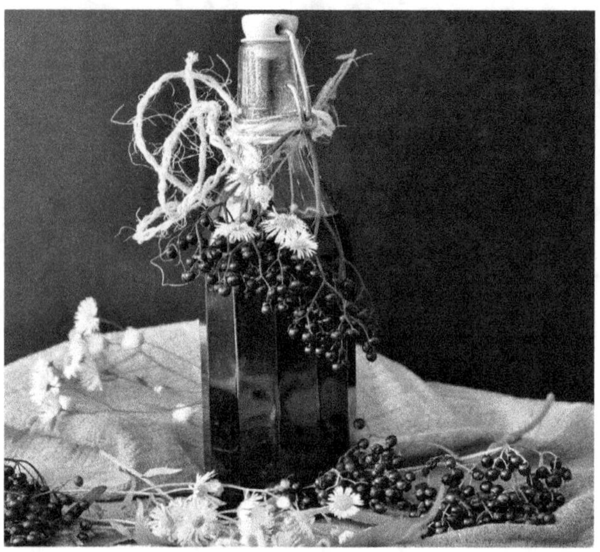

Ingredients:

- 1 cup dried elderberries

- 3 cups water

- Raw honey to taste

Directions:

Place elderberries in water in a large pot with berries covered with water at least 2 inches above elderberry.

Bring to a boil then immediately reduce heat to a simmer.

Continue to simmer until water is reduced to half its amount.

Remove from heat and let cool.

Pour into a blender and blend on low for a few seconds.

Strain with cheesecloth into glass jars and let cool.

Add raw honey to create the taste you desire.

Cover the jar with lid or top and shake until honey has dissolved.

Syrup lasts in the refrigerator for several months.

Herbal Elderberry Syrup

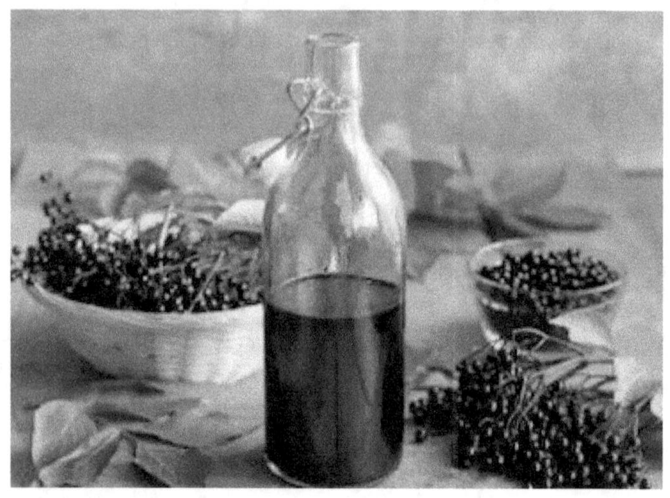

Ingredients:

- 1 cup dried elderberries

- 4 cups water

- 1 teaspoon ground cinnamon

- 1 teaspoon whole cloves

- 1 teaspoon ground ginger

- 1/4 cup wild cherry bark

- 1 Tablespoon dried orange peel

- 2 cups raw honey

Put all these ingredients into a sauce pan and bring to a boil on medium high heat.

Once the mixture boils, turn the heat down and let the mixture simmer for 30-40 minutes.

Using cheesecloth, pour the mixture into a large glass bowl.

Squeeze hard to get all the juice out.

Let the mixture cool a bit and add 2 cups honey to the mixture while it is warm, but not hot.

This makes about 5 cups of Herbal Elderberry Syrup. Syrup lasts in the refrigerator for several months.

Elderberry Compote

2 days to make to bring out the elderberry flavor

Ingredients:

- 1 lbs dried elderberries

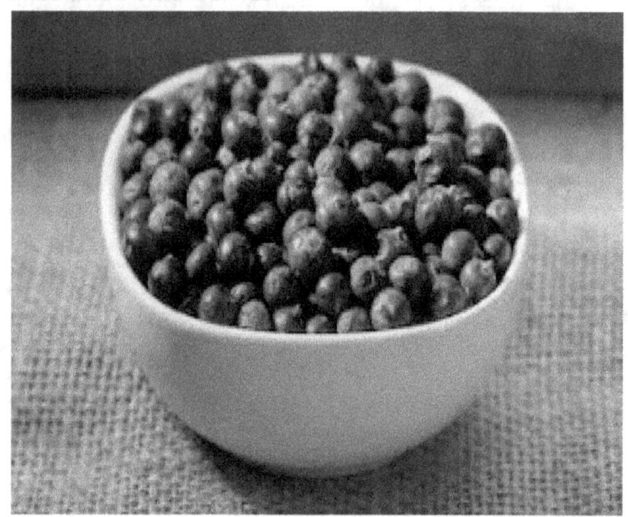

- 1 - 2 strips of lemon zest

- 1/4 split vanilla bean

- 1 - 1 1/4 cups raw honey or sugar

- 1/2 cup lemon juice

Directions:

In a glass bowl mix elderberry, lemon zest and vanilla bean.

Cover elderberry with honey/sugar and then cover with plastic wrap and set overnight.

24 hours later pour your mixture into a pot over medium heat.

Add lemon juice and bring to a boil, Immediately reduce heat to low.

If bubbling continues remove from heat entirely.

Pour into small glass jars leaving 1/2-inch space at the top.

Place jars in a hot water bath making sure jars are covered with water at least 1 inch.

Boil jars for 15 minutes.

Compote can store up to a year in a cool dark place.

Elderberry Vinegar

Can be added to things like barbecue sauce and salads.

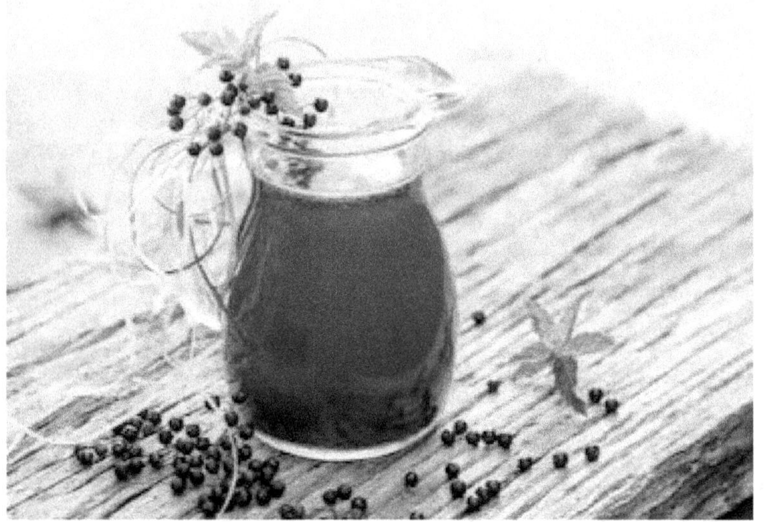

Ingredients:

- 2 cups dried elderberries

- 1 1/2 tablespoons sugar

- 2 cups 6% acidity white wine vinegar

Directions:

Mix the elderberries and sugar in a pan over medium heat.

Mash the elderberries while mixing.

Bring to a boil, immediately remove from heat and let cool.

Once completely cooled, mix berries and vinegar together and cover with plastic wrap.

Let sit for 3 - 5 days in a cool, dark place.

Strain through a cheesecloth thoroughly.

Store in a clean glass bottle.

Can be stored and used for up to two years.

Sparkling Elderberry

Energizing tart fruit drink with sparkling water

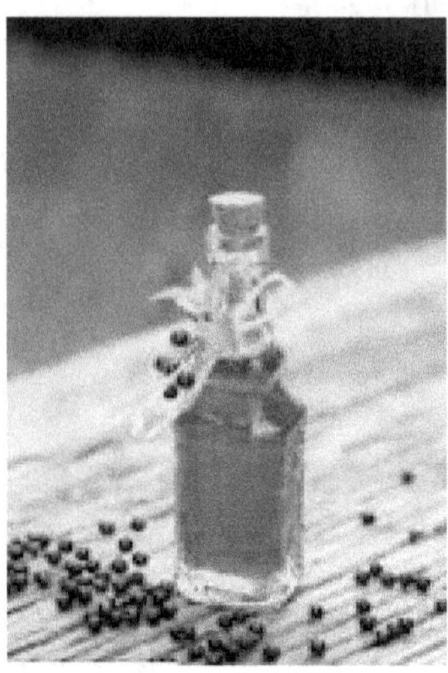

Ingredients:

- 2 cups dried elderberries

- ¾ cups raw honey or sugar

- 1 cup red-wine vinegar

- 1/4 cup water

- Sparkling carbonated water

Directions:

Pour the elderberries, sugar and water in a medium pot over medium heat.

Bring to a boil.

Once the honey/sugar is dissolved quickly turn down heat and simmer for 15 minutes.

Stir in vinegar and bring to boil again.

Turn down heat and simmer for 15 minutes again

Cool completely.

Strain through cheesecloth

Pour liquid into a glass cup, pressing on berries to extract all the juice.

Pour into clean glass bottle.

You can store for up to one year.

Pour a glass of Sparkling carbonated water and your Elderberry juice and enjoy whenever you want a cool refreshing drink.

Elderberry Custard

Make Elderberry Syrup first

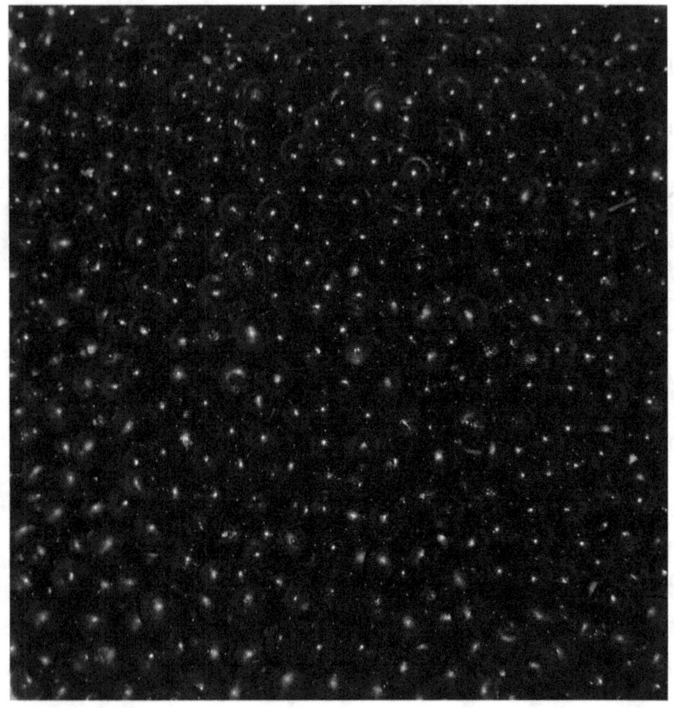

Ingredients:

- 2 cups heavy cream

- 1 - 2 tablespoons raw honey or sugar

- 1/8 teaspoon kosher salt

- 1/2 cup elderberry syrup

- Grated zest of 2-3 lemons

Directions:

Combine cream, sugar and salt and whip until cream peaks hold firm.

Gently fold in 1/2 cup of elderberry syrup all the while being careful to not lose the firmness of cream.

Divide among 6 - 8 glasses bowls and top with lemon zest.

Elderberry Elixir

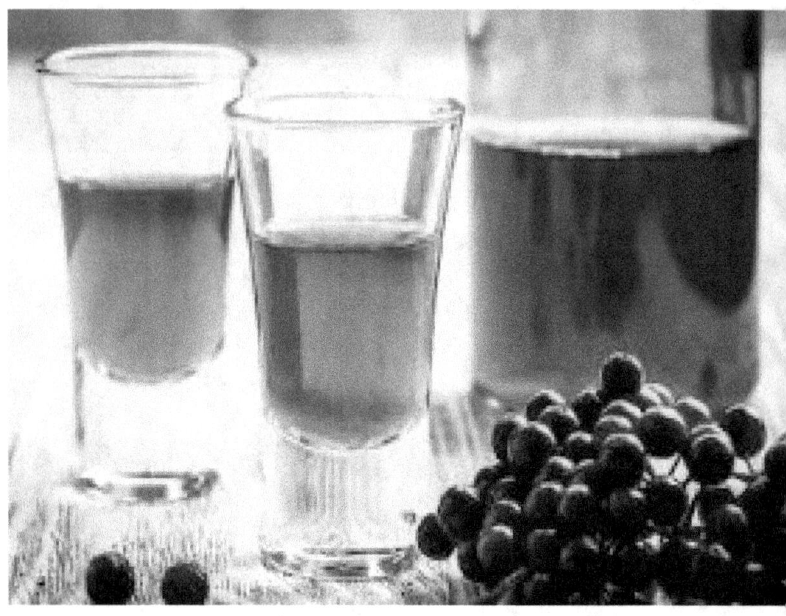

Ingredients:

- 2 cups elderberries

- 3 cups brandy or vodka

- 1 cup raw honey

Directions:

In a quart glass measuring cup fill ½ way with elderberries.

Pour alcohol to fill the jar ¾ full and then top with honey.

Stir the honey in with the berries until fully mixed.

Top off with more honey until the jar is full and stir again.

Close the jar.

Let sit for 3 weeks and shake daily.

After 3 weeks strain berries from the elixir.

Take 1 -3 teaspoons daily as it is said to help keep cold and flu away.

Elderberry Soup

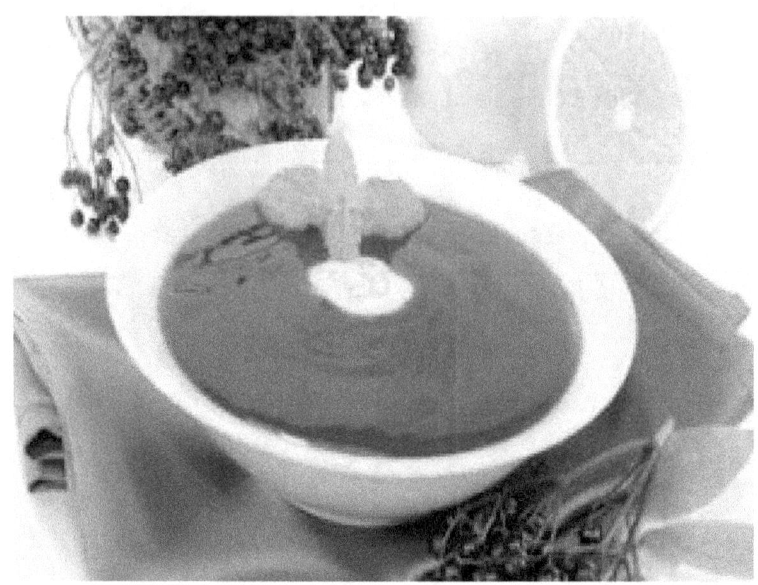

Ingredients:

- 1 cup dried elderberries

- 6 cups water

- ½ cup raw honey

- 1 tablespoon thickener like white flour or tapioca powder

- 2 tablespoons water

- 2 tart apples, peeled and diced

- 1 tablespoon grated lemon zest

- 1 tablespoon fresh lemon juice

Directions:

Bring the water to a boil over high heat. Add the berries and reduce the heat to medium. Cook until the berries begin to break down. Strain berries using cheesecloth and reserve the liquid and pour back into the cooking pot.

Add the apple cubes to the elderberry liquid and return to a medium heat.

Cook the apples until they are almost gone. Add back the strained berries, honey, lemon zest and lemon juice and simmer.

In separate pinch bowl mix the tablespoon of flour and 2 tablespoons of water thoroughly breaking any lumps. Slowly stir into hot soup. Simmer and stir for about 5 minutes as it thickens.

Serve. If you want cold soup chill for about 4 hours, then serve.

Elderberry Gummies

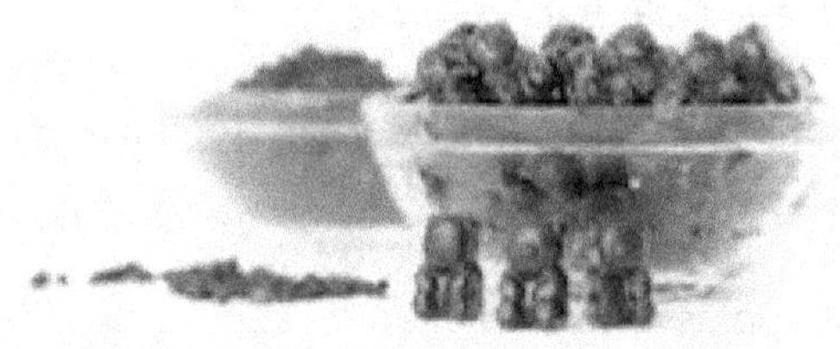

Ingredients

- 1 cup elderberry syrup (herbal or regular)

- ¼ cup gelatin powder

- ½ cup hot, not boiling water

- Silicone gummy mold

- Coconut oil

Instructions

Grease gummy molds with coconut oil to prevent sticking and set aside.

Place ¼ cup of cooled elderberry syrup in a glass bowl and using a whisk quickly whisk in the gelatin powder. Add the ½ cup of hot water and stir quickly and until smooth. Add the balance of the elderberry syrup and whisk until completely smooth. Pour into molds and refrigerate for 2 - 3 hours until completely firm. Pop out of molds and store in airtight container or glass jar.

To help prevent sticking very lightly dust with flour or coconut flour as desired.

Makes about 60 gummies

Elderberry Cordial

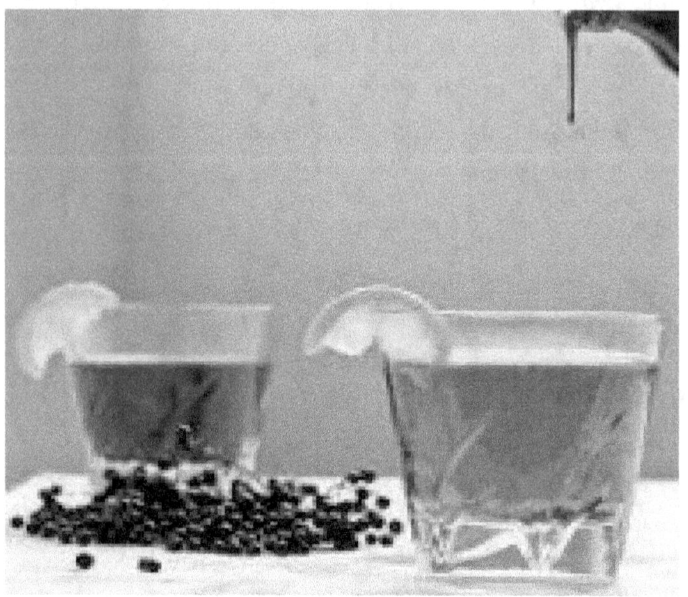

Ingredients:

- 1¼ cups dried elderberries

- 2 tablespoons minced fresh ginger or 1 tsp. dried 1 teaspoon crushed cinnamon

- 1/4 cup dried rosehips peel of one orange

- 2 ¾ cups water

- 3 cups Brandy

- 1 cup Raw honey

Bring all to boil then simmer for 10 minutes.

Allow to steep for an hour. Strain well through a couple of layers of cheesecloth

Then add 3 cups brandy and 1 cup Raw honey to taste.   Mix well.   Pour into jars cap and keep in a cool dark place.

Elderberry Lollipops

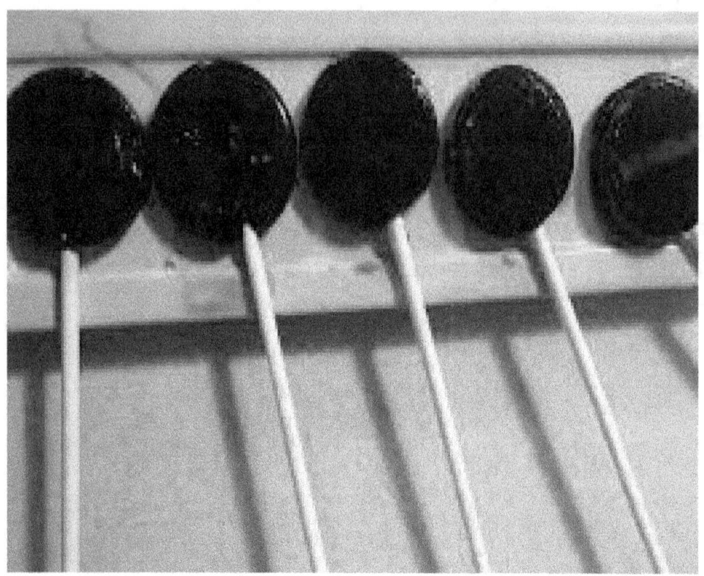

Ingredients:

- 1 tablespoon dried lavender cup fresh lavender

- 1 tablespoon dried lemon balm

- 1/2 cup elderberry syrup (choose Herbal or Basic above)

- 1 cup raw honey

- candy thermometer

- Silicone lollipop molds

Directions:

Brew the lavender and lemon balm with 1 cup water Bring to boil then simmer for 10-15 minutes then Strain.

Set lollipop mold on flat surface and place lollipop sticks in each of the molds.

Combined 1/2 cup of the strained tea, along with the elderberry syrup (Herbal or Basic) and honey, to a small saucepan.

Simmer on low, stirring frequently, when mixture starts trying to foam up stir constantly with a wooden or heat resistant spatula spoon while closely monitoring the temperature.

You want to reach 300 degrees, the hard-crack stage.

When the mixture reaches hard-crack stage remove pan from heat. Working quickly, pour into lollipop molds using soup spoon

Allow Elderberry Lollipops to rest undisturbed and still until fully cool and hard - about 30 to 45 minutes

Elderberry Jam

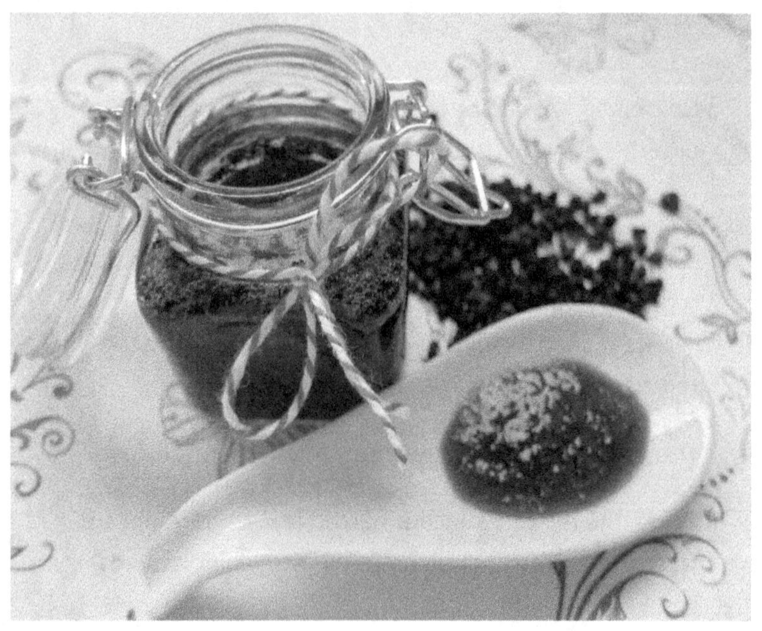

Ingredients:

- 2 cups dried elderberries

- 1 ½ cups honey

- 1 bag vanilla sugar

- juice of 2 lemon

- or 1 tablespoon lemon juice

Directions:

Soak elderberries overnight. Should yield 3 cups after soaking.

The next day place all the ingredients in a large pot. Stir so that the honey coats the berries. Cook until it boils and then continue to cook for another hourstirring often.

Remove from heat and let cool. Blend with hand mixer or use a wooden spoon to crush. Return to the heat and continue to cook until it thickens.

Elderberry Pie

This was one of the first elderberry recipes I began cooking with. When I first made elderberry pie I went out and gathered elderberries with the hummingbirds eating the berries right next to me. The hummingbirds were foraging faster than I was at times! The sensory memory of the hummingbirds zipping around me foraging is something that lives on in me to this day.

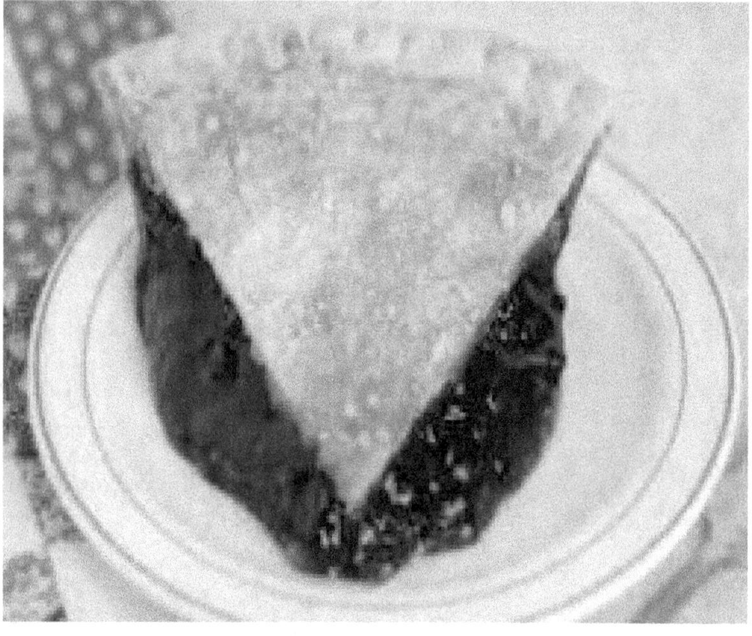

Talk about easy elderberry recipes, this pie is so very simple to make. You can go for straight elderberries or add in some apples for a great taste as well. Either way you'll come out with a rich and flavorful pie. Since most elderberries ripen towards the end of the summer, the dark colors of the elderberries contrasts with the fading colors of summertime.

For every cup of elderberries add in one tablespoon of melted butter and a teaspoon of arrowroot or cornstarch along with a hearty sprinkling of flour to serve as a thickener and to absorb the juice of the berries. Mix all this together in a bowl. If you want to add in apples then slice them up and fill your pie crust 1/2 to 3/4 full. Sprinkle with elderberries all over the apples.

Next in another bowl mix 1/2 - 1 cup of sugar with 2 - 3 tablespoons of flour and 1/8 teaspoon salt. Then sprinkle this on top. Now slice up and place a few tablespoons of butter on top of the pie. Bake at 450 for 15 minutes. After 15 minutes bake at 350 for 30 - 45 minutes until the crust is golden brown. One of my favorite wild foods radicals, Bradford Angier says that "the taste of elderberry pie when eaten in the perfumed breezes of the evening tastes pungently pleasant".

Elderberry Shrub

Elderberry shrub is a timeworn term for a tart fruit-based drink. The strong flavor of elderberries offers an energizing drink with sparkling water.

Ingredients:

- 2 cups elderberries

- 1/2 - 1 cup sugar

- 1 cup red-wine vinegar

- 1/4 cup water

- Sparkling carbonated water

Directions:

Pour the elderberries, sugar and water in a pan over medium heat. Bring to a boil. Once the sugar is dissolved immediately turn down heat and simmer 10 - 15 minutes. Stir in vinegar and bring to another boil. Turn down heat and simmer again for 15 - 20 minutes. Cool completely. Strain through a sieve or strainer. Pour liquid into a measuring cup, pressing on berries to pull out all the juice. Pour into clean glass bottle, jar or glass for drinking.

You can now either add sparkling carbonated water and enjoy fresh, or you can store in the refrigerator for up to one year and add sparkling carbonated water whenever you want to drink it. This is one of those elderberry recipes where the amount of sparkling carbonated water you mix with the volume of elderberry shrub is entirely up to your preference.

Elderberry Full Creamy

This recipe was originally a custard type dish (comprising of milk, eggs and sugar) and dates back to medieval times. Modern recipes have customarily replaced the custard for cream or pre-made whipping cream.

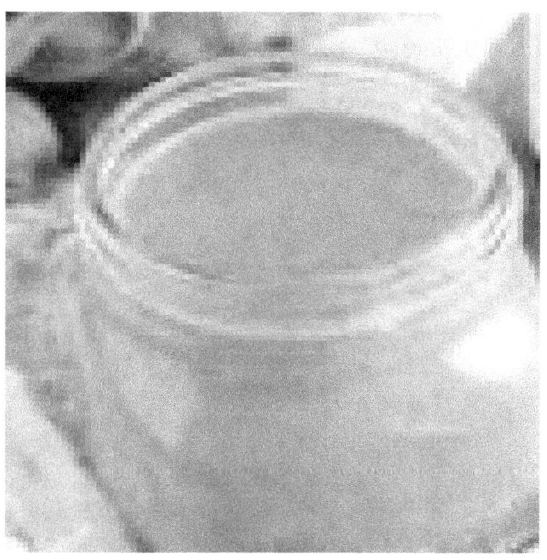

Ingredients:

- 2 cups heavy cream (raw cream is recommended)

- 1 - 2 tablespoons sugar (to taste)

- 1/8 teaspoon kosher salt

• 1/2 cup elderberry syrup or compote

• Grated zest of 1 - 2 lemons

Directions:

Combine cream, sugar and salt and whip until cream holds firm peaks. Gently fold in 1/2 cup of elderberry syrup/compote, creating a marbled effect in the cream all the while being careful to not lose the firmness of cream. Divide among 6 - 8 bowls or glasses and top with lemon zest. If you don't want swirls in your fool you can go with plain elderberries mixed in the cream instead of syrup or compote. Either way it's a teasingly delicious dessert.

Conclusion

What are the benefits of elderberry? For one thing, it has shown to seriously combat the common cold as well as the flu. Science has actually shown it can shorten flu symptoms by an average of four days.

Are elderberries poisonous to humans? No — there are actually many options when it comes to how you can consume elderberries, from juice to tea to jam. When taken properly, it typically has no negative side effects. In fact, researchers say its low cost, lack of side effects and clinical results make it an important tool for fighting flu.

One of the most popular ways to take elderberry, especially for a cold or flu, is a syrup, which is relatively easy to make at home.

Research is showing its potential ability to fight cancer, and hopefully more research is coming soon. It's also been shown to help lower blood sugar, ease allergies and improve cardiovascular health.

Elderberry has a pleasant berry flavor, and most people find it easy to take elder plant products.

Disclaimer

This book is not intended as a substitute for the medical advice of physicians. The reader should regularly consult a physician in matters relating to his/her health and particularly with respect to any symptoms that may require diagnosis or medical attention.

(HEALTH, ELDERBERRY)

About The Author

MY NAME IS DEZ SMITH

I am an entrepreneur who lives in the south with her kids and her Shiba Inu Max

I had the privilege of knowing my great grandmother for 35 years before her passing. She grew up in rural Augusta Georgia, farm country, where you took care of yourself helped your neighbors and trusted home remedies.

I often watched my great grandmother turn to different herbs for healing her mind body and soul before turning to prescription medication. As a child and young adult your opinions are formed sometimes without you knowing. But it was because of her that I to turn to herbal remedies before prescription medication.

I believe food is healing, herbs are healing and exercise strengthens the mind and body. I strive to instill these principles into my family so that one day each of us will have the privilege of knowing our great grandchildren.

I really love educating people on how to stay healthy and live the life of their dreams.

Do not go yet; One last thing to do

If you enjoyed this book or found it useful I'd be very grateful if you'd post a short review on it. Your support really does make a difference and I read all the reviews personally so I can get your feedback and make this book even better.

Thanks again for your support!